Copyright

Johanna Kristin Ellerup, PharmD

Contributing Editor: Olga Kalugina, PharmD

2019
Johanna Kristin Ellerup PharmD
All rights reserved.

ISBN: 9781706804864

No part of this book may be reproduced, or stored in a retrieval system, or transmitted in any form or by any means, electronic, mechanical, photocopying, recording, or otherwise, nor in any language without the express written permission of the author.
Printed in the United States of America

TABLE OF CONTENTS

DIABETES	**4**
Epidemiology and Generalized Information:	4
Recommendations	4
Patient Counseling points:	5
Cover terms	7
Clinical Pearls & Notes:	9
Signs and symptoms of associated disease states:	11
Pathophysiology:	13
Treatment options:	16
Lifestyle Interventions –	17
DPP-4	18
GLP-1	22
Alpha-Glucosidase	28
Meglitinides	30
Sulfonylureas	32
First generation agents	32
Second Generation	32
Sodium Glucose Transporter Protein2 – Inhibitors	35
Thiazolidinediones	38
Biguanides	40
Amylin Analog	43
Insulin	45
Anti-Hypoglycemic Agent/Glycogenolytic	53
Clinical Guidelines:	55
References:	55

Diabetes

Epidemiology and Generalized Information:
Prevalence 1.25 million Americans. Incidence is 40,000 new diagnoses each year.

2013 – 33-49% of patients not meeting general targets for glucose

33-49% of patients not meeting general targets for glucose, BP or cholesterol & only 14% met goal while not smoking.

2012-17 – cost of diabetes (w/adjustments for inflation) increased 26%

Social determinants of health are economics, environment, political & social conditions in which people live.

14% of Americans suffer from food insecurity & increased risk of T2DM, suboptimal glycemic control, psychosocial conditions and low treatment adherence [79].

Recommendations

A—Clear evidence from well-conducted, generalizable randomized controlled trials that are adequately powered

B—Supportive evidence from well-conducted cohort studies

C—Supportive evidence from poorly controlled or uncontrolled studies

E—Expert consensus or clinical experience

- BMI - >=25Kg/m2 or >=23 Kg/m2 in Asian Americans. Consider testing [Level B recommendation]
- Everyone gets tested at 45 years of age [B]
- Repeat testing, if normal and conditions listed, roughly every 3 years [C]

- In patients w/pre-diabetes & T2DM – test & if needed treat for cardiovascular issues [B]
- Pre-diabetes risk screening in children or adolescents who are overweight (BMI >=85%) [B]
- Patient centered, open-ended positive response, collaborative health care team approach. [B]
- Multidisciplinary team with interactive communication [E] [79]

Patient Counseling points:

1) Do not double doses. If close to the time of the next, subsequent dose, skip the dose you missed and continue regimen. Consider making a note (i.e., in diabetes diary) of missed dose to reconcile any blood glucose fluctuations.
2) Swallow tablets/capsules whole. Do not crush or chew.
3) Store all injectables out of direct sunlight. Refrigerate, do not freeze, prior to use and maintain within acceptable room temperature once vial is punctured or pen is utilized.
4) Do not shake injectables; instead hold between both palms and gently swirl.
5) Use alcohol swabs to clean vials and skin prior to puncturing and rotate injection sites to reduce injection site reactions and lipodystrophy.
6) Report any unusual or elevated reactions or side effects to your doctor immediately. If in doubt, call 911.
7) Carry identification somewhere on your person at all times indicating that you are diabetic for emergency purposes.
8) Keep portable candies and long acting carbohydrates/protein on hand and utilize mobile apps for guidance.
9) Contact your provider during illness as physiologic needs may change.
10) Notify all providers of medical history, including history of gallstones, ethanol, smoking, pancreatitis,

hepatic/renal disease, cholesterol level and current medications including Over-the-Counter items, herbals and supplements.
11) Check all vials and pens (where possible) for cloudiness, changes in color or particulate matter. Dispose of safely in sharps containers.
12) Unless otherwise stated in the package insert, cloudy insulins (glargine, isophane, etc.) should not be given intravenously.
13) Vials follow ISMP (Institute for Safe Manufacturing Practices), US Pharmacopeia standards of 28 days stability after puncturing a multi-dose vial unless otherwise stated in the package insert.
14) Those with diabetes should check their feet routinely and protect from cuts, corns, blisters and injuries that may compromise skin integrity. Diabetic patients are more prone to fungal and bacterial infections of the extremities, especially if they suffer from diabetic neuropathy which can decrease awareness. Suggest they make a habit of doing a quick, yet thorough, inspection while changing their socks, shoes. IF the patient notices any changes to their feet or calves, advise them to notify their primary care physician, podiatrist and/or dermatologist immediately.

Cover terms

Fasting Blood Glucose (FPG) – Macrovascular disease – Metformin, Insulin. Fasting – greater than 6 hours between meals – 70-100 (up to 130)

Post-Prandial Glucose (PPG) and A1C – Microvascular disease – GLP-1, DPP4, Insulin & SGTP. Peak postprandial – (peak – 1-2 Hrs after **initiation** of meal) = <=180mg/dl.

Preprandial – Similar to trough – just prior to eating 70-130

HbA_1C – Normal non-diabetic patients 4-6%. Very strict control is <7. Some patients may require <8 to prevent hypoglycemia.

Primary failure – Inability to achieve disease remission/optimal effect with evidence based drug treatment and doses.

Secondary effect – After initial success, the agent loses effectiveness which may be neutralization by pathogen enzyme secretion, alternate pathway or irreversible over-saturation of receptors (down regulation).

75g oral glucose tolerance test (OGGT) – With either fasting plasma glucose (FPG) or 2HR plasma glucose.

The 2Hr plasma glucose diagnoses, overall, more patients than either the FPG or A_1C.

Diagnosis requires, at least, two elevated and separate test results (even A1c) unless there's obvious signs of hyperglycemia – 3P's – polyuria (urine), polyphagia (eating) & polydypsia (drinking), etc. Repeat testing in 3-6 months.[8] This distinguishes transient hyperglycemia (temporary alteration in diet, infection, drug treatment, etc.) from diabetes.

Pre-diabetes – Not a clinical diagnosis, but rather a warning to increase monitoring and non-pharmacologic pathways. [8]

Pediatric and geriatric patients display altered pharmacokinetic/dynamics and therefore require different treatment, dosing or increased monitoring. Start low and go VERY slow. For example, pediatrics have different Vd and an immature GI tract/hormone secretions, so that a drug may have greatly reduced serum levels or have a higher level excreted unchanged. Geriatrics may have greatly reduced renal or hepatic function not fully evident on labs, so that the duration of action of a 6 hour tablet that undergoes second pass effect may be increased to 24 plus hours in this patient population.

The 'Incretin Effect' is defined as the insulin response difference in oral versus IV dosing of glucose. A possible explanation for this increased effect, in some cases a three-fold increase, is the digestive enzyme secretion in saliva. By the time food has entered the stomach via the lower esophageal sphincter, the pancreas has been actively stimulated in preparation whereas an IV injection bypasses this mechanism.

Under normal conditions, glucagon is secreted by the alpha cells of the Isle of Langerhans, which also secretes beta and delta cells, of the pancreas in response to fasting conditions and maintains glucose concentration within the plasma. Insulin is secreted by the beta cells of the Pancreas, in response to meals and stimulates the uptake of glucose to peripheral tissue and out of the plasma circulation thereby reducing solutes in plasma.[31]

Clinical Pearls & Notes:
Categories of diabetes: Think - 3P's – Poly-urea (urinating/micturating), Poly-dypsia (drinking), Poly-phagia (eating). Think – increased osmolarity (dissolved particles in solute) of blood for pathogenesis of primary and secondary disease.

All agents that induce the secretion of insulin can lead to pancreatitis.

Genetic missense variants: Known pathogenicity in the *GCK (highly overrepresented in DM)*, *HNF1A*, *HNF4A*, *ABCC8*, and *INS* genes.[11]

DNA amino acids: G (guanine), T (thymine), C (cytosine), A (arginine).

SNP – Single Nucleotide Polymorphisms – change to one specific nucleotide in an open-reading frame that may alter the translation/transcription of that sequence.

T1DM = Immune mediated or idiopathic – AKA Juvenile Diabetes.[8]

T2DM = Insulin resistance peripherally w/relative insulin deficiency or more commonly effect on insulin secretion with insulin resistance. AKA adult diabetes. In this class, hyperglycemia may follow metabolic syndromes = obesity, HTN, hyperlipidemia & impaired fibrinolysis. (AHFS,3211)

HbA_1C – "…nonexzymatic glycosylation of other proteins throughout the body as a result of recent (eg. previous 6-8 weeks) hyperglycemia." (AHFS, 3212)

Microvascular complications include blindness, retinopathy, and nephropathy rely, co-morbid with dyslipidemia, blood pressure and vascular thrombosis. Most associated with PPG. AHFS

Agents that have CYP 450, OAT/OCT, PgP interactions, etc – even when 'not clinically significant' may play an important role to individual patients displaying unexpected sides or reactions. Don't dismiss them.

Agents that are excreted in bile and/or unabsorbed from the GI tract is eliminated in feces. Consider this if agent affects GI transit time or binds to the GI tract excessively.

In general, the insulin or sulfonylurea dose is reduced preferentially over DPP-4, GLP-1 or SGTP.

Beta blockers, hypothyroid agents, anxiolytics, catecholamines agonists/antagonists may mask hypoglycemic signs and alter glucose metabolism.

Insulin is preferred in pregnancy and pediatrics due to increased Vd, decreased muscle and altered adipose tissue. In general, oral agents are reserved for 18+.

Geriatric patients (70+) have reduced renal, hepatic and cardiac function and therefore, in general, may use lower dosages or increased intervals with all agents to reduce hypoglycemia which can lead to falls, dizziness, altered mental status, etc.

Insulin is needed in ketonuria and glucosuria.

Hypoglycemia treatment protocol – IV D50W 50mL Bolus with D10W titrated to glucose >100mg/dl. Glucocorticosteroids, such as dexamethasone, may be added.

Signs and symptoms of associated disease states:

Hepatic Failure: ALT/AST >120 (3 times upper limit of normal [ULN]); elevated Alk Phos (indicative of liver, bone disease), yellowing of sclera, skin (jaundice), abdominal pain, nausea, vomiting, fatigue, anorexia, dark urine, ascites.

Pancreatitis: Serum & urine amylases increased, amylase/CrCl ratio, electrolyte imbalance, sCa^{2+}, glucose and lipase.

Thyroid Tumors: Malignant or benign, lump on base of neck that (key characteristic) bobs up and down with swallow mechanism (follows thyroid), hoarseness, dysphagia, dyspnea). Prevalence ~ 6% female, 1-2% male. Up to 95% are benign, but must be evaluated. Consist of cysts, goiter (commonly in hypothyroid), adenomas and nodules. [57]

Lactic Acidosis: Fatigue, headache, mental instability, increased lactase dehydrogenase and liver function tests (LFT's).

Metabolic Acidosis: Tachypnea, anorexia, nausea, vomiting, lethargy, mental status changes and abdominal pain.

Diabetic ketoacidosis: Blood glucose levels needn't be >200, but an increased anion gap, elevated blood and/or urine ketones, mental status changes may be present. Potential factors include hypovolemia, acute renal failure, hypoxemia, reduced oral intake, ethanol ingestion, acute illness (infection) and reduced insulin dosage.

Renal labs: Hgb/Hct, electrolytes, BUN/sCr, CBC. Signs: Increased water retention (edema), HTN/hypotension, unconcentrated urine, skin turgor, appetite changes, digestion alterations, addition of NSAIDs, ACEI, diuretics, digoxin, etc.

Fournier Gangrene: Necrotizing fasciitis, tenderness, swelling, redness of genitals, back to the rectum, 100.4+ fever, malaise, increased LDL-c hypoglycemia.

Alcohol consumption in Diabetes – Alcohol displays varying effects depending on fed/fasting state of patient and whether acute or chronic ingestion. It can increase blood glucose in the fed state, due to a reduced inhibition (I.e., person may consume more carbohydrates calories), the sugar content of the drink itself, an alteration in fat metabolism, and an increase in peripheral insulin resistance. Whereas in chronic or starvation states the depletion of glycogen and alcohol preventing hepatic gluconeogenesis can cause blood glucose levels to plummet to dangerously low levels. This is compounded by the fact that hypoglycemia awareness is blunted during alcohol consumption and, due to the above listed events, there is an attenuated response to correction of hypoglycemia.[80]

Pathophysiology:

1) **Type 1 Diabetes** – Polygenic form. Attributed to several genes, including HLA-DQA1, HLA-DQB1, and HLA-DRB1 genes contribute 5% toT1DM population. HLA is human leukocyte (white blood cell) antigen (a pathogenic cell). Considered auto-immune – where immune cells are attacking Isle of Langerhans-Pancreatic Beta Cells that secretes insulin. Pancreatic alpha-cells secrete glucagon.[16]
   Signs – 3P's, unexplained weight loss, excessive fatigue.
   Signs of DKA – "Sweet fruity breath" – Hallmark feature, dry or flushed skin (also thyroid or CHF), stomach pain (variety, including liver, bowel obstruction, etc), disoriented, SOB.
   Number 1 treatment is insulin replacement.
   Several agents- DPP4, GLP-1, Sulfonylureas, Meglitinides- are not compatible with T1DM because they stimulate the secretion of insulin from the pancreas which is the key feature separating Type 1 from Type 2. Hence, the side effect of pancreatitis for these agents.[13]

2) **Type 2 Diabetes** – Polygenic form. Think – overuse/over-stimulation disease. *IGF2BP2* -SNP rs4402960 (Insulin-like growth factor 2 mRNA-binding protein 2; single Nucleotide Polymorphism) G/T, TERT rs2735940 T/C, TERT rs2736098 G/A.[15] T2DM is also associated with Metabolic Syndrome (hypercholesterolemia, hyperglycemia, hypothyroidism, hypertension), which doesn't rule out an inflammatory disorder. Evidence shows that the DASH and Mediterranean diets may have positive outcomes.
- This is the only type of diabetes that is amenable to diet and exercise alone.
   Signs – 3P's, increased fungal infections, sores that don't heal (may also indicate cancer, psoriasis, etc).

3) **Diabetes Insipidous** – Polygenic form. "Sweet Urine." Insipidus – (think – insipid) light and odorless. Normally, adults pass approximately 1-2 quarts (1/2 gallon, app 1890ml) of urine daily. DI patients can pass up to 20

quarts (app 5 gallons) of unconcentrated urine, due to an abnormality in renal tubular filtering. Important difference - Normal blood glucose levels (normoglycemic).

Four major types of DI:

a. ***Centrally mediated*** – Hypothalamus or pituitary. Vasopressin, a vasoconstricting agent that increases plasma sodium leading to increased water retention and increased blood pressure, does not concentrate the urine. Causes include central trauma, infection, meningeal inflammation, etc.

b. ***Nephrogenic*** – Adrenally mediated. Vasopressin does not concentrate urine. BUN/sCr can be utilized to discern whether there is pre-renal implications (blockage), lithium and other exogenous xenotropic causes, altered electrolyte status.

c. ***Dipsogenic*** – Excess fluid intake, especially water. An altered mental or physiologic status that causes more fluid intake than the body can normally process, thereby unfiltered excretion of the excess. Causes include all those previously listed.[18]

d. ***Gestational*** – Transient. May be caused by prostaglandin or oxytocinase/vasopressinase that inactivates vasopressin. Treatment of choice is DDAVP (desmopressin) that mimics the effects of vasopressin without inactivating or attenuating oxytocin (Pitressin – used to reduce pre-term labor).[19]

4) **Gestational Diabetes** – Treatment is insulin, as transport of oral agents across the placenta, risk of hypoglycemia and their varied side effects on the developing fetus is controversial at best. Co-morbid diseases include pre-eclampsia (very elevated blood pressure that is dangerous to both the mother and fetus), enlarged baby (possible developmental and/or physiological disorders),[20] At-risk mothers - age >35,

previous gestational diabetes or primary family member, previous high birth weight delivery, pre-pregnancy obesity, hormonal disorders (ie., Polycystic Ovarian Syndrome). May be managed with non-pharmacologic factors and insulin. If uncontrolled, infants have a higher pre-disposition of developmental disorders (learning disabilities), heart disease, hyperlipidemia and diabetes later in life.

5) **Monogenic Diabetes Syndromes** – A form of non-autoimmune, early onset diabetes that arises from a variant in one gene. It accounts for 1-4% of all DM cases in the US. May or may not be germline or a spontaneous mutation.[11, 12]
   a. Neonatal – May be transient, occurring only as the neonate begins to mature, or may be lifelong. Occurs in ~1 out of 400,000 US infants. Key determinant is that T1DM is rarely seen before 6 months of age, but NDM exists at birth. May also appear slightly later, ie toddler onward.
   b. Maturity Onset Diabetes of the Young (MODY) – A monogenetic disease that is heritable. Historically, these patients have chronically elevated blood glucose, but not necessarily peripheral or end-organ disease or overweight. Diagnosed via genetic testing. Medications are not necessarily preferred in this patient class.

6) **Secondary Diabetes**: Exocrine Pancreas (cystic fibrosis, pancreatitis, etc), Drug/Chemical induced, neonatal diabetes (non-NDM form), etc.

Treatment options:

Diabetes Diary: Recommend the utilization of a diary to all patients, regardless of history or acumen in managing their diabetes as a method of tracking their glucose measurements and treatment.

- Suggest online diaries for tech savvy or highly active patients. A wide variety, 'MyNetDiary', 'GlucoseBuddy', *et al* exist.

Non-Pharmacologic in T2DM

Diet – complex carbohydrates produce longer AUC of glycemic effect with less peak/trough fluctuations

Exercise/Lifestyle interventions – Improves mobility of glucose to peripheral tissues and blood circulation/perfusion.

Pharmacologic:

Insulin – ALL types of DM. First line in T1DM. May be initiated at any point in T2DM, given patient acceptance of injections.

Metformin – First line [FPG, PPG, 2HR, micro & macrovascular] – prophylaxis, BMI >=35, aged < 60 years, women with gestational diabetes mellitus, polycystic ovary disease, amenorrhea.

Remaining agents are for T2DM:

Second line – DPP-4, SGLT or GLP-1 [PPG, HbA_1C & microvascular]

Third line – Sulfonylureas/Thiazolidindiones

Fourth line – Meglitinides (Cardiac sides)

Fifth line – alpha-glucosidase [PPG, A_1C & microvascular]

Lifestyle Interventions –

a) Utilize DASH diet and Diabetes Prevention Program to get BMI (Body Mass Index) within limits & increase physical activity to, at least, moderate intensity (brisk walking) activity at least 150 min per week.
b) Diabetes Prevention Program outcomes – diabetes reduced 58% over 3 years. Follow-up: sustained reduction in rate of conversion to T2DM of 34% at 10 years and 27% at 15 years.
c) Also, Alternative Healthy Eating Habits Index (AHEI): whole grains, legumes, nuts, fruits & vegetables, and decreased intake of processed or refined foods.
d) Foods that will reduce the risk of diabetes – nuts, berries, yogurt, coffee & tea.
e) Foods that increase the risk of diabetes – red meat & sugared beverages

Important - Plasma glucose usually 10-15% higher than in whole blood.[8]

DPP-4
AHFS 2016, 3205-3216

FPG, PPG, A_1C, micro & macrovascular.

Mechanism of Action: Glucagon-like peptide (GLP-1) and glucose-dependent insulinotropic peptide (GIP) inhibits the secretion of glucagon and hepatic glucose production via signaling mechanisms that include cAMP (cyclic adenosine monophosphate). Dipeptidyl-peptidase -4, expressed in the GI tract, liver, kidneys, endothelial vascular beds, etc., inhibits GLP-1 and GIP, leading to decreased insulin secretion.[34] Theoretically, agents that directly affect these molecules (DPP-4, GLP-1 & GIP) are glucagon dependent, therefore there's a lower incidence of hypoglycemia than other agents.

Effective for both PPG and FPG – so will reduce risk of micro and macrovascular disease.

SAVOR-TIMI 53 – found that saxagliptin increased hospitalizations for acute heart failure, but no increase in cardiovascular events. DPP-4's - EXAMINE – found no increase in cardiovascular events in ACS patients. TECOS – no significant increase in cardiovascular events.[33] May be acceptable in cardiac patients – EKG and regular monitoring suggested. All agents that stimulate the secretion of insulin from the pancreas carry a risk of pancreatitis. Bullous Pemphigoid development is a serious immune reaction that requires discontinuation of this class of agents.[35]

<u>Class sides</u>: Pancreatitis, abdominal pain, nausea, vomiting, arthralgia, hyperlipidemia, hypertriglyceridemia, reduced renal function, angioedema, urticaria, pruritus, reduced lymphocytes, hypoglycemia, anaphylaxis, upper respiratory infection, headache, nasopharyngitis.

Sitagliptin (Januvia): <u>Package Insert</u>

Available – 50mg & 100mg
REMS was rescinded.
HbA_1C reduced by 0.5-0.7%.
No adjustment needed in Child-Pugh <=9.
Renal dosing adj: CrCl 30-45mL/min = 50mg QD.
    < 30mL/min = 25mg QD.
Vd:198L. F:87%. $T^{1/2}$: 12.4 Hr. Cl: 350mL/min. Peak: 1-4 Hrs.
Protein Bound: 38%
Elimination: 13% in feces, 87% in urine.
Metabolised 3A4, 2C8, OCT (Organic Cation Transporter), P-glycoprotein (PgP).

Saxagliptin (Onglyza): <u>Package Insert</u>, <u>Medscape</u> [1] & <u>DrugBank.ca</u> [54]

Available – 2.5mg & 5mg.
Biphasic metabolism due to 50% active metabolite 5-hydroxyl-saxagliptin.
HbA1c reduced by 0.5%.
No adjustment needed in Child-Pugh <=9.
Renal dosing adj: CrCl 50mL/min or 3A4 inhibitor=2.5mg QD.
Vd:Negligible. F:87%. $T^{1/2}$: 2-2.5Hrs. 5-OH= 3.1 Hrs. Cl: 151L/min. Peak: 2 Hrs, 5-hydroxy-saxagliptin = 4hrs. Protein Bound: 67%
Elimination: 22% in feces, 75% in urine.
Metabolised 3A4, 3A5, PgP. Of note: Chelates cations (Mg^+, Al^+, Ca^{2+}).

Linagliptin (Tradjenta): Package Insert & DrugBank.ca [58]

Available – 5mg QD. Xanthine derived DPP-4 inhibitor (Allopurinol, smoking).
HbA$_1$C reduced by 0.4-0.5%. Weight reduced ~1.1Kg (although weight gain is possible).
No adjustment needed in Child-Pugh or renal ***.
Vd: 1110L. F:30%. T$^{1/2\ biphasic\ elimination}$: 100 Hr. Cl: 374mL/min.
Peak: 1.5 Hrs. Protein Bound:75-89 % (reduced binding at higher concentrations).
Elimination: 90% in urine.
Metabolised 3A4, OCT (Organic Cation Transporter), P-glycoprotein (PgP), aldo-keto & carbonyl reductases. CD1790 is predominant metabolite.

Alogliptin (Nesina): AHFS & DrugBank.ca [55]

Available – 12.5mg & 25mg
HbA$_1$C reduced by 0.55-0.6% (56).
No adjustment needed in Child-Pugh <=9.
Renal dosing adj: CrCl 30-60mL/min = 12.5mg QD.
    < 30mL/min = 6.25mg QD.
Vd:417L. F:~100%. T$^{1/2}$: 21 Hr. Renal Cl: 9.6L/hr, Cl: 14L/hr..
Peak: 2-3 Hrs. Protein Bound: 20%
Elimination: 13% in feces, 76% unchanged in urine.
Metabolised 3A4, 2D6. Minimally Metabolised. One active metabolite (N-demethylated Alogliptin <1%) and one inactive (N-acetylated Alogliptin <6%). 99% exists as R-enantiomer.
NOTE: Heart & Hepatic failure associated with this agent.

*** Even though these agents alter renal and hepatic AUC or peak alterations, they have not been demonstrated to be clinically significant, so dosage adjustments are not indicated. Bear it in mind however, for patients that display alterations due to illness, addition of medications or other morbidity.

GLP-1
AHFS, Pgs: 3216-3230

PPG, A$_1$C & microvascular. **Not First Line.**

GLP-1 receptors are located in cerebral ventricles and hypothalamus (temperature regulation). Associated with appetite satiation.[32]

Glucagon-like peptide-1 is produced when pro-glucagon is cleaved post-translationally and secreted in two active forms, GLP-1 (**7**,36) and GLP-1 (**7**,37), two inactive forms **9**,36 and **9**,37, and shortened by the dipeptidyl peptidase-4 (DPP-4) enzyme cleaving the second proline or alanine on the N-terminus[22], by L-type cells of the small intestine. GLP-1 is also found elsewhere, such as the hindbrain preproglucagon neurons[23] and mediates gastric motility, stimulates Isle of Langerhan beta cell proliferation, differentiation and apoptosis inhibition[25], which stimulates insulin secretion and suppresses glucagon secretion. Pre-proglucagon neurons are activated via cholecystokinin (CCK) and leptin, both of which are satiety peptides, whereas ghrelin, an orexin peptide, doesn't. Also, the central amygdala is associated with hunger and satiety. This area, and numerous others including microglia is known to have GLP-1 receptors and to be modulated by IL-6 downstream, possibly providing further explanation for the hypophagia and reduced inflammatory effects of agents utilizing this mechanism. [24,25]

The inflammatory process is directly correlated to the initiation and progression of diabetes, so agents that alter that process indirectly affect glucose uptake and metabolism. This is most commonly evidenced by the elevation of serum glucose with corticosteroids and HMG-CoA reductase inhibitors.[26,28,29]

Serotonin 5HT-2a, which causes hypophagia, reduction in body fat and overall weight loss, and 5HT-2c expression is altered with GLP-1 agonism.[30] Delays in gastric emptying is also attributed to this process and agents that affect this receptor, either directly or indirectly. Elevations in cAMP, via the Glucagon-

Protein Kinase A pathway, leads to increased depolymerized glucose production.

These agents, in addition to at least two other agents, exhibit a two-fold risk of gall bladder and bile duct disease possibly attributed to the up-regulation of cholangiocytes.[39]

Class Effects Summarized: Saeity, wt loss, increased insulin secretion via reduced glucagon release, decreases GI emptying also attenuating glucagon release with no impairment on normal glucagon regulation. Increases 3',5' cAMP to increase insulin release in presence of elevated glucose. Also, vasodilatory effects and anti-inflammatory effects. Take all medications 1 hour before or 4 hours after these agents.

Class Side Effects: Pancreatitis, hypoglycemia, reduced renal function, GI (N,V, D), antibody production, anaphylactic reactions (urticaria, pruritus), autonomic reactions (jitteriness, hyperhidrosis, dizziness, headache, etc) GERD, Hashimoto's thyroiditis, constipation, upper respiratory tract infection, urinary tract infection, back pain.

Contraindicated: Medullary thyroid carcinoma, multiple endocrine neoplasia syndrome and monitor in Hashimoto's.

Liraglutide: Victoza. Saxenda approved for weight loss. **AHFS & DrugBank** [59]

The peptide precursor is 97% analogous to endogenous, active GLP-1(**7**,37) which makes up less than 20% of circulating GLP-1. The endogenous arginine 34 is replaced with a lysine and the lysine at 26 is attached to palmitic acid with a glutamic acid spacer to form Liraglutide.

Available – 0.6mg – 1.8mg. Starting dose 1.2mg injection.
Saxenda = 3mg.
REMS due to C-Cell Cancer. Must register patients with manufacturer maintained C-Cell cancer registry.
HbA_1C reduced by 1.1%. Wt loss ~3Kg.
Vd:13L. F:55%. $T^{1/2}$: 13 Hr. Cl: 1.2L/hr. Peak: 8-12 Hrs. Protein Bound: 98%
Elimination: 5% in feces, 6% in urine.
Metabolised 3A4, 2C8. Remainder to CO_2 and H_2O.
Storage in refrigerator (2-8°C) when unused and at room temperature <=25°C after. Discard pen after 30 days. Do not use if particulate matter, color change or cloudy. Never double doses. Inject subcutaneously in thigh, upper arm or abdomen. For minor injection site reactions, cold compress, antihistamines or NSAIDs may be utilized with advice from primary care provider only.

Exenatide: Byetta, Bydureon. AHFS & Drugbank.ca [60]

Available – 5mg – 10mg BID Byetta. Bydureon 20mg QW 1 hour before a meal.
REMS due to pancreatitis & medullary thyroid carcinoma.
HbA1c reduced by 0.7-0.9%. Wt loss ~3Kg.
CrCl: <30ml/min – do not use.
Vd:28.3L. F:1%. $T^{1/2}$: 2.4 Hr. Cl: 19.1L/hr. Peak: 2 Hrs. Protein Bound: Unknown
Elimination: Proteolytic glomerular cleavage and filtration with elimination in urine.
Metabolism: 3A4
Created from the saliva of the Gila monter with a 53% similarity to endogenous.

Lixisenalide: Adlyxin. AHFS & Package Insert[82]

Available – 10mcg SQ QD for 14 days then may up-titrate to 20mcg
HbA$_1$C reduced by 0.7%. Wt loss neutral. FPG reduced ~14.
CrCl: <30ml/min – do not use.
Vd:100L. F:100%. $T^{1/2}$: 3 Hr. Cl: 35L/hr. Peak: 1-3.5 Hrs. Protein Bound: Unknown
Elimination: Proteolytic glomerular cleavage and filtration with elimination in urine.
It consists of a 44 amino acid (aa) peptide that amidated at the C-terminus of aa#44 in a string-like (open chain) configuration.
NOTE: angioedema (bradykinin).
Each Green 50mcg/ml (3ml) pen = 15 days or 7.5 days at maintenance dose.
Each Burgundy 100mcg/ml (3ml) pen = 30 days or 15 days at maintenance dose.

Dulaglutide: Trulicity. AHFS & Package Insert [83]

Available – 0.75mg QW & 1.5mg QW in 3ml pens.
REMS: C-Cell Carcinoma and Thyroiditis.
HbA_1C reduced by 0.7-1.6%. Wt loss ~3.4Kg.
CrCl: <30ml/min – do not use.
Vd:19.2 & 17.4 (1.5mg)L. F:56%. $T^{1/2}$: 5 days. Cl: 0.109L/hr.
Peak: 48 Hrs. Protein Bound: Unknown
Elimination: Proteolytic glomerular cleavage and filtration with elimination in urine.
Fusion protein containing 2 disulfide chains that is covalently linked to the Fc of a human-modified IgG4 heavy chain via a peptide linker produced in a mammalian cell culture ([61]).
The amino acid sequence is 90% homologous to endogenous human active GLP-1 (7,37).

Semaglutide: Ozempic. AHFS & Package Insert [62]

Available – 0.5mg or 1mg QW
Starting dose is 0.25mg QW for 4 weeks then 0.5mg QW for 4 weeks. May increase to 1mg QW after 4 weeks.
HbA_1C reduced by 1.5%. Wt loss ~5.6Kg. FPG reduced 29mg/dl. PPG reduced 74 mg/dl.
CrCl: <30ml/min – do not use.
Vd:12.5L. F:89%. $T^{1/2}$: 7 days. Cl: 0.05L/hr. Peak: 1-3 days.
Protein Bound: >99%
Elimination: Proteolytic glomerular cleavage and filtration with elimination in urine.
Important note: Semaglutide will be present in plasma for up to 5 weeks after discontinuation.
Peptide backbone is produced via yeast fermentation.
Semaglutide's long half-life is due to albumin binding, modification of position 26 lysine with a hydrophilic spacer and a C18 fatty di-acid, modified in position 8 to provide stabilization against degradation by DPP-4 & position 34 to ensure the attachment of only one fatty di-acid.

Albiglutide: Tanzeum. AHFS & Package Insert[63]
Name: Think two tandem copies.
Available – 30mg SQ QW; can increase to 50mg QW SQ.
Package contains 4 pens with 29gauge 5mm thin wall needles.
Pens expire 8 hrs after reconstitution,
REMS: Medullary thyroid cancer.
Increased incidence of afib/aflutter – patients were male, older,pre-existing renal impairment or cardiac disease at baseline.
Average increase in heart rate was 1-2 BPM.
HbA_1C reduced by 0.8-1%. Wt loss ~0.6Kg.
No dosage adjustment in renal or hepatic insufficiency.
CrCl: <30ml/min – do not use.
Vd:11L. F:Unknown. $T^{1/2}$: 5-7 days. Cl: 67mL/hr. Peak: 48 Hrs.
Protein Bound: Unknown
Elimination: Proteolytic glomerular cleavage and filtration with elimination in urine.

Directions for use:
It is a lyophilized powder contained in a pen. There must be 4+ days between doses in dose titration. Can take a missed dose up to 3 days later, otherwise skip.
The diluents and lyophilized powder is mixed by holding the pen upright so the #1 appears in the window. The clear cartridge on the pen is twisted in a clockwise fashion till the #2 'clicks' into the window.
Do not shake.
Tilt the pen back and forth gently or side-to-side 5 times to mix, then let it sit for 15 min (30min for the 50mg) pen to ensure the mixture is homogenized.
Prior to administration – tilt the pen again 5 times, check the window for yellow, clear of particulates, solution and inject it within 8 hours.
Holding the pen upright, attach the needle to the pen by pushing it straight down until a 'click' is heard and the needle snaps into place.
Recombinant fusion protein where 2 copies of modified human CLP-1 is fused in tandem to human albumin using S. Cerevisiae. The human GLP-1 (**7**,37) is changed – glycine is substituted for alanine-8 in order to be able to resist DPP-4 proteolysis.

Alpha-Glucosidase

AHFS 2013, pgs. 3147-3151

PPG, A_1C & microvascular.

Approximately 1/3 is excreted in urine.[3]

Not to be used with SGTP (Sodium Glucose Transporter Protein Inhibitor) agents.

Inhibiting alpha-glucosidase on the lumenal side of the small intestine, leads to a decrease in GI transit time, reduction in available circulating glucose and a reduction in the elevation of post prandial glucose.[4] This also leads to the side effects of increased flatulence – increased glucose stasis.[4] Found in the brush border of the enterocytes of the (small) intestine and pancreatic alpha-amylases located in the lumen. Pancreatic alpha amylases digest complex starches to oligosaccharides and sucrases, maltases and isomaltases hydrolyze oligo, tri and disaccharides into glucose, etc.[5]

- Acarbose cannot be hydrolyzed, due to its imino bridge by these digestive enzymes. Acarbose is metabolized by intestinal digestive enzyme cleavage and biotransformation by intestinal microorganisms.[5]
- Not unlike mannitol or glycerin suppositories (sugar alcohols, etc) increase in glucose in the intestines increases the interaction with bacteria and yeasts leading to alterations in GI colonization and sides such as flatulence, bloating, abdominal pain, diarrhea, etc.[4,6]

Alpha-glucosidases are maltase-glucoamylase and sucrose-isomaltase. Each enzyme is composed of 2 subunits on the C and N termini of their proteins. All 4 (2 on each terminal) can hydrolyze maltose & only 2 (C terminal end) can hydrolyze sucrose. Some agents that may have similar MOA include Black Currants, Rowanberry, Cinnamon Bark and possibly black tea so caution in patients taking these supplements.[7] Glucosidases include, but not limited to, alpha glucosidase, B glucosidase,

Cellulase, Maltase, debranching enzyme. Reduction of FBG 0.7% and 1% HbA$_1$C.

Class side: Pneumatosis Cystoides Intestinalis – radiologically mimics necrotizing enterocolitis gas filled vesicles in the intima lining of the Jejunum, ileus or cecum (duodenum).

Acarbose (Precose) <u>AHFS 2013</u>

Eliminated in bile. C25H43NO18 mw-645.6
Available: 25-50mg QD and increase over months to 50mg TID if <=60kg or 100mg TID >=60kg.
Reduction of FBG 0.7% and 1% HbA$_1$C.

Miglitol (Glyset) <u>AHFS 2013</u>
Eliminated renally (sugar alcohol) 95% Negligible protein binding. C8H17NO5. MW-207.224
Duration 4-6 hours; max dose – 300mg; $T^{1/2}$ – 2.7-9Hr.
Reduction of FBG 0.7% and 1% HbA$_1$C.

Meglitinides
AHFS 2013, Pgs. 3210-3218

Warning – Cardiac sides – Starlix
Class Action Summary: "Closes ATP-dependent K^+ channels in the Beta cell membrane by selective binding – this causes depolarization which opens Ca^{2+} channels the resulting increased Ca^{2+} influx induces insulin secretion." (4, 9) Also, binds to the Sulfonylurea receptor (adjacent to the SU binding loci) and stimulates release of insulin from beta cells. Release is glucose dependent (4).

Gender effects (possibly 3A4) - 15-70% increased AUC in females but disappeared when data normalized for dose and weight. So, it appears that women are started on this drug at a higher BMI requiring a higher dose, therefore more potential for negative sides, than men.

Class sides: Musculoskeletal, headache (hepatically derived? Or CYP3A4) Paresthesias, pain, hyperesthesia, dizziness and fatigue, UTI (micturation), allergy, tooth disorder, increased appetite (3A4 histamine), WT again, rash, increased Liver enzymes, thrombocytopenia and leucopenia hemolytic anemia, alopecia, pancreatitis, SJ syndrome, severe hepatic dysfunction (jaundice & hepatitis).

Class Effect: Short-acting secretogues (4). Mutations in CYP2C9, CYP2C8, SLCO1B1, SLC30A8, NEUROD1, PAX4, KCNJ11, KCNQ1, TCF7L2, and NR1I2 negatively affect response to meglitinides.[21]

Nateglinide (Starlix) AHFS

2C9 & 3A4. $T^{1/2}$ – 1 H Duration – 4H. 120mg TID. Weakly active 3A4.
Renally eliminated metabolites
D-Phenylalanine derivative – **phenylketonurics.** Those unable to metabolize increased doses or with other agents (like sugar free items) increases dopamine and norepi – leading to increased cardiac effects.

Repaglinide (Prandin) AHFS

Available: 0.5-1mg TID Max 16mg QD.
$T^{1/2}$ 1Hr. Duration 4Hrs. 3A4 inactive metabolites. Bile excretion. Reduces HBA_1C – 0.6-1%
Total body CL – 38L/hr; Plasma Cl 33L/Hr; linear correlation dose & plasma – Zero order kinetics. 90% excreted feces (2% as Rep); 8% in urine (0.1% as Rep) Peak: 1.5hrs post-dose. Dur: 4 Hrs.

Majority metabolized as dicarboxylic acid = 60% of metabolism. 3A4 and 2C8 via oxidation, dealkylation to major dicarboxylic acid derivative (M2) and further oxidation to an aromatic amine derivative (M1). An acyl glucuronide metabolite (M7) formed from the COOH group of repaglinide. Also binds to alpha-glycoprotein and albumin.
Severe renal (CrCl 20-40ml/min) = 0.5mg TID and increase carefully

Sulfonylureas
AHFS, Pgs. 3268-3287

NOTE: Aside from insulin, this may be the most thoroughly researched class of medications.

Binds to B cell membrane at ATP dependent K^+ channel to close them – depolarization and opening of voltage gated CA^{2+}. Increases intracellular CA^{2+} leads to increased insulin secretion.[4; pg 1343]

First generation agents
Will be included for historical or reference only, as they are no longer in general use owing to either increased side effects or longer duration leading to severe hypoglycemia.

Acetohexamide, Chlorpropamide – SIADH (one treatment agent demeclocycline) hyponatremia dose dependent; cholestatic hepatitis, Tolazamide, Tolbutamide – dose dependent SIADH.

Second Generation
Reduced dosing as prolonged $T^{1/2}$ leads to accumulation in elderly. As opposed to first generation, all second generation are non-competitive, non-ionic protein binding.

Class sides: Severe hypoglycemia, SJS, disulfiram (more 1st gen), pancreatitis, diarrhea, gastralgia, constipation, eczema, tremor, pyrosis, pruritus, neuropathy, weight gain, anaphylaxis, fever, jaundice, anemia, sulfa allergy, G6PD hemolytic anemia, cardiac (edema like DPP-4 & meglitidines), SIADH (less than First gen), dysgeusia, hemolytic instability (40, 41). Vision changes become more vital to monitor if the patient is also taking digoxin, a fluoroquinolone, etc.

Glimepiride (Amaryl) [40,41]

Available – 2mg average dose. 8mg Max. 1-4mg QD or BID.
HbA$_1$C reduced by <2% Weight reduced ~1.9Kg.42
Vd:8.8L. F:100%. T$^{1/2}$: 4-6 Hr. Cl: 47.8mL/min. Peak: 2-3 Hrs.
Protein Bound:99.5 %
Dur 18-28Hrs.
Elimination: 60% in urine; 40% feces.
Metabolised Hepatically 2C9, 3A4
Metabolized via oxidative biotransformation to weakly active (M1) cyclohexyl hydroxyl methyl via 2C9 while keeping 1/3 the pharmacologic effect. M1 is metabolized in the cytosol to M2, which is inactive.[43]

Glipizide (Glucotrol) (45 & AHFS)

Available: 2.5-5mg initial the increase. If >10mg consider BID. Max 40mg

HbA$_1$C 1%. Weight increased 0.6Kg
Vd: unknown. F:80-100%. T$^{1/2}$: 10 Hr. Cl: 374mL/min. Peak: 1-3 Hrs. Protein Bound:92-9 % . Renal Cl: 21-38 L/hr.
Elimination: 60-90% in urine.
Metabolised 2C9, 3A4.

Converting from insulin to glipizide:
Insulin <= 20 units – 2.5 -5mg tablet
Insulin >= 20 units – decrease Insulin by 50% and start with 5-10mg glipizide (AHFS).

Inhibits platelet aggregation (serotonergic effect) induced by collagen or ADP (adenosine Diphosphate), which may or may not be clinically significant. Monitor all patients on SSRI's, trazodone, NSAIDs, ASA, DOACs, ulcers, increased risk of GI, bleed or stroke.[45]

Glyburide (Micronaze, Diabeta) ([44](), [45](), & [AHFS]())

Available – micronized 1.5, 3, 5, 6mg – max 12mg. Regular 1.25, 2.5, 5mg – max 20mg.
HbA_1C reduced by 1.9% Weight increased ~2 Kg
Vd: 9-10L. F:100%. $T^{1/2}$: 4 & 10 Hr. Cl: 78L/Hr. Peak: 2-4Hrs.
Protein Bound:99 %
Dur: 18-24Hrs
Elimination: 50% in urine, 50% in bile/feces.
Less active metabolites 4-trans-hydroxyglyburide & 3-cis-hydroxyglyburide (most active).
Metabolised 3A4.
Glyburide also produces mild diuresis, so monitor with mannitol, diuretics, NSAIDs, reduced oral intake and SGTP agents.
The ACCORD trial – HbA_1C reduced 1% and ~2 Kg weight gain.[45]

Converting from insulin to glyburide:
Insulin 20 units – 2.5 -5mg tablet
Insulin 20 - 40 units – 5mg
Insulin > 40 units - decrease Insulin by 50% and start with 5mg glyburide & titrate at 2 week intervals.[AHFS]

Sodium Glucose Transporter Protein2 – Inhibitors
AHFS 2016, Pgs. 3258-3268

Class sides: UTI – including pyelonephiritis and urosepsis, vaginal pruritus, increased micturation, nasopharyngitis, back pain, thirst, renal, weight loss, dehydration, ketoacidosis, mycotic infections - **Fournier gangrene** of the perineum, hypotension, bone fractures, increased LDL and anaphylaxis.

All undergo hepatic second-pass effect.

Not in pregnancy.

Mechanism of Action: Selectively inhibits re-absorption of glucose in the proximal renal tubule, therefore glucose concentrates in the urine (Think creating diabetes insipidus). Monitor with dehydration states, diuretics, ACEI/ ARB's, mannitol, iodinated contrast medium, NSAIDs, and all agents that can cause electrolyte abnormalities, dehydration or renal insufficiency.

Uridine glucuronosyltransferase (UGT) inducers include rifampin, phenytoin, phenobarbital, ritonavir and others.

This class of drugs can paradoxically increase endogenous glucose production to maintain osmolarity and hemodynamics (AHFS).

Ertigliflozin (Steglatro) Package Insert & AHFS

Available – 5-15mg PO QD.
HbA$_1$C reduced by 0.7%. Weight decreased ~2 Kg
Vd: 85.5L. F:100%. T$^{1/2}$: 24 Hr. Cl: 11.2L/Hr. Peak: 1Hrs. Protein Bound:93.6%
Elimination: 50.2% in urine, 40.9% in bile/feces.
Not recommended in eGFR <30 mL/min or severe hepatic disease (Child-Pugh C).
Metabolised 3A4. UGT1A9 and UGT 2B7 mediated o-glucuronidation to 2 inactive glucuronides, whereas oxidated metabolism is 12%.
Ertigliflozin is a substrate of P-glycoprotein (P-gp) and breast cancer resistance protein (BCRP) transporters.

Dapagliflozin (Farxiga) Package Insert

Available – 5-10mg PO QD.
HbA$_1$C reduced by 0.8%. Weight decreased ~4.4 Kg
Vd: unknown. F:78%. T$^{1/2}$: 13 Hr. Cl: 11.2L/Hr. Peak: <2Hrs. Protein Bound:91%
Elimination: 75% urine, 21% feces (15% as parent drug).
Not for eGFR <60mL/min or severe hepatic disease (Child-Pugh C).

Specific side – increased risk of bladder cancer and extremity pain.
Dapagliflozin 3-O-glucuronide is substrate of OAT3 (Organic anion Transporter) and a weak PgP substrate.

Empagliflozin (Jardiance) Package Insert

Available – 10mg & 25mg PO QD.
HbA$_1$C reduced by 0.7%. Weight decreased ~3 Kg FPG = -30
Vd: 73.8L. F: Unknown T$^{1/2}$: 12.4 Hr. Cl: 10.6L/Hr. Peak: 1.5Hrs.
Protein Bound:86 %
Elimination: 54.4% in urine, 41% in bile/feces.
Not for eGFR <45mL/min or severe hepatic disease (Child-Pugh C).
Undergoes glucuronidation to 2-O-, 3-O-, and 6-O-glucuronide metabolites – UGT 2B7, 1A3, 1A8 and 1A9, OAT3, 1B1, 1B3. Substrate only, not inhibitory. Substrate of BCRP and PgP.

Canagliflozin (Invokana) Package Insert

Available – 100mg & 300mg PO QD.
HbA$_1$C reduced by 0.8%. Weight increased ~3.4 Kg
Vd: 83.5L. F:65%. T$^{1/2}$: 10.6 & 13.1 Hr. Cl: 192mL/min. Peak: 1-2Hrs. Protein Bound:99 %
Elimination: 30% in urine, 41.5% in bile/feces.
eGFR 60-45mL/min use 100mg; NOT recommended in eGFR<45mL/min.
O-glucuronidation is the major metabolic elimination pathway for canagliflozin, which is mainly glucuronidated by UGT1A9 and UGT2B4 to two inactive O-glucuronide metabolites. CYP3A4-mediated (oxidative) metabolism of canagliflozin is minimal (approximately 7%) in humans.

Thiazolidinediones
AHFS 2016, Pgs. 3287-3296

Mechanism of Action: Increased insulin sensitivity, peripheral glucose uptake, a decrease in hepatic gluconeogenesis via peroxisome proliferator-activated receptor2 (PPAR2) agonism that increases the transcription of insulin.[48, AHFS, pg.3291]
Do not directly stimulate the release of insulin.
Greater detail: "Altered free fatty acid influx to skeletal muscle and regulation of adipose differentiation leading to the production of small, compact and more insulin sensitive fat cells with decreased epinephrine receptors...increased adiponectin and decreasing free fatty acids and TNF-alpha."[46]
"Weight gain might be edema...reduced renal excretion of Na+ and altered intestinal ion transport or microvascular permeability secondary to enhanced production of VEGF."[46]

Class sides: Hypoglycemia, fluid retention, cough, fatigue, increased LFT's, hepatitis, bone loss (osteopenia), non-vertebral bone fractures (distal forearm/hand, knee/foot), bladder cancer, ovulation induction (due to peripheral sensitization to glucose), macular edema, visual changes (monitor with other agents that affect vision, like digoxin), anemia, increased CPK (creatine phosphokinase) and CK (creatine kinase), upper respiratory tract infection, headache, jaundice.
The weight gain class effect may be due to an increase in subcutaneous fat as a result of lipogenesis from improved insulin sensitivity combined with the peripheral edema.[45, AHFS]

Pioglitazone (Actos) Package Insert & Drugbank.ca

Available – 15mg & 30mg PO QD. Max 45mg QD.
HbA_1C reduced by 1%. Weight increased ~3.6 Kg
Vd: 0.64L. F:65%. $T^{1/2}$: Pio 3-7, metabolites (M3 & M4) 16-24 Hr. Cl: 6L/Hr. Peak: 2Hrs. Protein Bound:99 %
Elimination: 15-30% in urine, remainder possibly in bile/feces.
Metabolism – CYP450 2C8 (gemfibrozil, rifampin, etc), 3A4.
Primarily first pass hydroxylation and oxidation & the metabolites M3 & M4 also partly convert to second pass glucuronide or sulfate conjugates.
There is an increased AUC and Cmax of 20-60% in females.
Reduced Trigs, increased HDL, no change in LDL or Total Cholesterol.

Rosaglitazone (Avandia) Package Insert & AHFS

Available – 2 & 4mg PO QD or BID. Max dose = 8mg
HbA_1C reduced by 0.8-1%. Weight increased ~2.8 Kg. FPG – reduced 35-40
Vd: 17.6L. F:99%. $T^{1/2}$: 3-4 Hr. Cl: 3L/Hr. Peak: 1Hrs. Protein Bound:99 %
Elimination: 68% in urine, 23% in bile/feces.
No renal adjustment but reduce dose in Child-Pugh B/C.
Reduces fatty acids/Trigs ~10%, increases LDL & VLDL ~ 16%, increases HDL ~14%.
Major side – worsening of congestive heart failure. FDA removed REMS in 2016.

Biguanides

Metformin (Glucophage)
Package Insert & AHFS 2016, Pgs. 3190-3204

Available – 500mg, 750, 1000mg PO QD & BID. ER = 500mg, 850mg, 1000mg.
Max dose = 2.5Grams. Note: Some may not see effect till 1.5G dose.
HbA$_1$C reduced by 1.5%. Weight neutral. FPG – reduced 35-40
Vd: 654L. F:50-60%. T$^{1/2}$: 6-9 Hr. Cl: 491mL/min. Peak: 2-4Hrs.
Protein Bound: Equilibrates between plasma and erythrocytes
Elimination: Triphasic elimination as unchanged drug.
For use in T1DM and T2DM. Reduces microvascular and macrovascular risk.
Metabolised renally and secreted by proximal renal tubules. Hold for 48 hours prior to and after iodinated contrast material due to renal effects of each.
Contraindicated in renal (sCr >1.4mg/dL) and hepatic disease.
Reduces fatty acids/Trigs ~10-15% and TotChol 7%, increases LDL & VLDL, increases HDL.

Mechanism: Reduces both fasting and postprandial via sensitizing peripheral tissue to insulin, thereby reducing hepatic gluconeogenesis and enhancing glucose oxidation. Also, enhances insulin stimulated activation of GLUT1 and GLUT4 to the plasma membrane of the peripheral target cells like skeletal muscle and adipose tissue.
May effect tissue plasminogen activator in some patients, so monitor is NSAIDs, ASA, DOACs, warfarin, clopodogrel, etc.

Derived from guanidine (Galega officianalis), which is a dimethylbiguanide. The dimethyl increases H$_2$O solubility and decreases binding to mitochondria, plasma membranes, etc. This was an issue with the agent phenformin.

Sides: Nausea, vomiting, diarrhea, flatulence (GI effects because it binds to intestinal wall), GERD, bloating, metallic taste, constipation, anorexia, decreased B12, headache, dizziness, HTN, musculoskeletal pain. Most resolve spontaneously.

Lactic acidosis – symptoms to monitor for include malaise, dizziness, increased somnolence, respiratory distress, bradyarrhythmias, mental status changes possibly due to tissue hypoperfusion, hypoxia.
   Labs: lactate dehydrogenase >45mg/dL, pH less than 7.35, abnormal electrolytes, increased anion gap, increased lactate/pyruvate (measure of anaerobic activity) ratio.[AHFS]

Drugs that alter renal function include alcohol, steroids, statins (also increase blood glucose levels), sympathomimetics, Ca^{2+} blockers, isoniazid, ACEI/ARBs and lithium, to name a few.

Metformin is also used for PCOS – Polycystic ovarian syndrome. Insulin resistance, elevated blood glucose, metabolic syndrome, achronic anovulation (oligomenorrhea or amenorrhea), hyperandrogenism with clinical manifestation of irregular menstrual cycles, infertility, hirsutism, obesity, acne and dyslipidemia.
Metformin increases oocyte maturation and release possibly associated with increased glucose uptake and insulin sensitivity, therefore used to induce fertility.

Caution:
All diuretics will decrease plasma volume and increase glucose levels. Monitor patients carefully, especially in cases of volume-depleting co-morbidities such as diarrhea, vomiting, or adjunct agents such as SGTP agonists.
Several agents such as B-blockers, Calcium channel blockers, catecholamine agonists/antagonists, hypothyroid agents, can mask the signs of hypoglycemia. B-blockers also worsen glucose tolerance, alter hemodynamic response to hypoglycemia and, due to a reduction in cardiac output, they may impair peripheral circulation. Nonselective, non-ISA agents may be better. These

agents block epinephrine, which has anti-insulin/pro-glucagon effects, increases peripheral tissue uptake of glucose, decreases free fatty acids thereby enhancing muscle uptake of glucose.[67]

Amylin Analog

Pramlintide (Symlin)
Package Insert & AHFS 2016, Pg.31898-90

For PPG, microvascular. Use in T1DM and T2DM.
Available – 1.5ml Symlin 60, 2.7mL Symlin 120.
HbA_1C reduced by 0.4%. Weight increased ~1.3Kg. FPG – reduced 35-40
F:30-40%. $T^{1/2}$: 48 min. Peak: 1Hrs. Protein Bound: Not significant
Elimination: Renal. No adjustment in renal insufficiency. Approximately 40% unbound in plasma.

Mechanism of Action: Its action doesn't alter the regulatory response to hypoglycemia.[AHFS] Acetate analog of human amylin with substitution of proline at Alanine25, Serine 28 and serine29. Amylin is secreted from the same Islet of Langerhans Beta cells that secrete insulin. Like insulin, there is a reduced secretion in diabetes. Amylin reduces gastric emptying, suppresses glucagon secretion, which reduces hepatic gluconeogenesis and induces centrally mediated appetite suppression.

Major sides: Hypoglycemia and gastroparesis, nausea, vomiting, anorexia, headache, dizziness, arthralgia, fatigue and injection sight reactions. The hypoglycemia may be severe due to the fact that this is an adjunct to insulin.

Caution: Due to the heightened risk of severe hypoglycemia and gastroparesis with this agent any patient that is at a risk for non-compliance, pediatric, geriatric, those with reduced GI motility (surgery, opiates, etc), has a history of hypoglycemia or hypoglycemia unawareness should not take this agent.

Counseling:
Do not mix with insulin. Protect from light. Refrigerate, do not freeze. Once used, only for 30 days.
Do not inject in the arm due to variable absorption. Only thigh or abdomen, rotating sites.
Meals must contain >=250kCal or >=30 grams of carbohydrate.
Visibly inspect for color changes, particulate matter prior to injecting.
Take medications, especially those with a narrow therapeutic window like digoxin & thyroid agents, 1 hour before or 2-3 hours after injections.
    Reduce the insulin dose by 50% prior to initiation.
    Wait at least 3 days prior to up-titrating dosages.
    T1DM = 15mcg SQ before meals to a max of 60mcg.
    T2DM = 60mcg SQ before meals to a max of 120mcg.

Insulin
Package inserts, AHFS 2016, Pgs. 3230-58

PPG, A1C & microvascular

Calculating the insulin dose can be found here[69]

Basal insulin initiated at 10units/HS. HS dosing needed due to peak plasma glucose occurring in AM due to symogyi effect. Carbohydrate calculation for regular insulin injection based on average diet.

Action	Insulin	Kinetics
Basal	Glargine – Lantus, Basaglar, Toujeo (300U/mL)	Onset: 1Hr Peak: 2-20Hr Dur: 24
	Detemir - Levemir	Onset: 1-2Hr Peak: 3-9Hr Dur: 6-24
	Degludec - Tresiba	Onset: 1Hr Peak: 9Hr Dur: 24+
Rapid	Lispro - Admelog	Onset: 15-30min Peak: 30min-2.5Hr Dur: 3-6.5Hr
	Aspart - Fiasp	Onset: 15-20min Peak: 1-3Hr Dur: 3-5 Hr
	Glulisine - Apidra	Onset: 20min Peak: 45-50min Dur: 4-5.5Hr
Intermediate	Lispro – Humalog	Onset: 1Hr Peak: 30-90Min Dur: 6
	Protamine Lispro – Humalog 75/25; 50/50	Onset: 30min-1Hr Peak: 1-6Hr Dur: 13-22
	Isophane and	Onset: 30-90min

	Insulin (rDNA) 70-30 – Humulin 70-30 (70)	Peak:3.5Hr Dur: 18-24
	Aspart – Novalog (contains Protamine & Zinc)	Onset: 10-15 min Peak:1-3Hr Dur: 3-5 Hr
	Neutral Protamine Hagedorn (NPH) and Regular – Novolin NPH 70/30	Onset: 1-3Hr Peak:6-8Hr Dur: 16-24
Regular	Novolin R, Humulin R	Onset: 30-60Min Peak:1-5Hr Dur: 6-8 Hr

Guidelines: Note: Guidelines may change slightly, but these are the standard goals.

Insulin administration should mimic endogenous insulin secretion as closely as possible, therefore 3-4 injections daily is common. Of these, 1 is basal – preferably at bedtime to counteract morning glucose increase, followed by 2-3 daily post-prandial injections. Monitoring with test strips should be done 3-5 times daily. Common regimens are long-acting basal injections at bedtime followed by 2 intermediate injections during the day to reduce number of painful injections. Additional goals include individualizing all patients care, but especially those with co-morbid conditions. Insulin resistance may require increased doses and can be seen in patients taking anti-psychotics, steroids, with infections, trauma, endocrine abnormalities, etc.

Critically ill hospitalized patients should be maintained at 110-140mg/dL FBG to reduce mortality.

Preschoolers and adolescents have a higher rand, FPG 100-180 and over night of 110-200 with a target HbA_1C of 7.5-8, due to their immature regulatory systems, GI alterations and hypoglycemic unawareness. Adolescents and young adults have FPG 90-130, overnight PG levels of 90-150 and HbA_1C of <7.5. Non-diabetics have an HbA_1C of 4-6 & FPG 70-100.

Insulin doses = 0.2-1 Unit/Kg pre-prandially with 40-60% of the dose given as a long-acting basal.

The basal is dosed at 0.1-0.2 Units/Kg or a flat 10Units at bedtime to start, then increased 4 units every 3 days as needed to reduce hypoglycemia.

To calculate the patients initial insulin requirement, utilize the many online website such as this, taking into account the patients activity level, any diet changes, co-morbid diseases and basal energy expenditure if needed.

Normally given subcutaneously with alcohol pads, 28-31 gauge needles, 1.3-1.6mm in length ('pen needles'), appropriate diabetic testing machine, any control solutions, and testing strips.

Side effects: Dyspnea, hypotension, tachycardia, urticaria, pruritus, angioedema, diaphoresis, which are hypersensitivity reactions that may be caused by circulating insulin antibodies. These reactions occur less frequently in human derived insulin than in the bovine or porcine products. Other sides include hypertrophy, lipodystrophy, hypokalemia as insulin shifts potassium intracellularly & erythema at the site.

Treatments utilizing insulin: High dose insulin is utilized in calcium channel and beta-blocker overdoses[73] possibly due to its ability to shift calcium intracellularly, positive inotropic effects, prevents anaerobic consumption of a stressed heart by providing glucose, cAMP effects increase circulation and perfusion to overcome the reduce cardiac output of beta blocker therapy, and may reduce the insulin resistance of calcium channel blocker therapy.[74] It is also utilized to reduce the hyperglycemic states caused by disease, enteral nutrition therapy, shock, medications (glucocorticosteroids, diuretics, protease inhibitors, etc). It is the preferred treatment option in pregnancy.

Agents that directly counter insulin include, but are not limited to, glucagon, estrogens, somatotropin, epinephrine, levothyroxine, triiodothyroxine, thyroid stimulating hormone, vasopressin and aldosterone.[75, 76, 77]

Only skeletal, cardiac and adipose tissue require insulin transport. Insulin facilitates the hepatic phosphorylation of glucose-6-phosphate to glycogen, stimulates lipogenesis, inhibits lipolysis, protein synthesis and release of free fatty acids from adipose tissue.

Somogyi Effect vs Dawn Phenomena –

Somogyi Effect – A rebound hyperglycemic event where counter-regulatory hormones and transmitters (growth hormone from the anterior pituitary, cortisol, glucagon and epinephrine) in response to elevated insulin dose (hypoglycemia). Usually only effects T1DM. Treatment is a complex carbohydrate at bedtime and to reduce the bedtime insulin dose.

Dawn Phenomena – Generally occurs around 3AM due to growth hormone release. This is NOT a rebound effect, but rather simply elevated glucose. Treatment is to increase bedtime insulin dose or administer it closer to bedtime and reduce evening snack.

Metabolism: Insulin is rapidly metabolized by hepatic glutathione, insulin transhydrogenase, renal and muscle tissue. The kidneys filter insulin and 98% is reabsorbed in the proximal tubule. 40% is returned to venous flow and 60% is metabolized within the proximal renal tubule itself. The Cl is 1.23L/Hr. It consists of an alpha chain and a beta chain joined by disulfide bridges.

Aspart – Rapid acting. Saccharomyces Cerevisiae.[84] B chain alterations: 28 Proline substituted with 28 Aspartic Acid.

Glulisine – Rapid Acting. B Chain alterations: 3 Asparagine becomes lysine; 29 Lysine becomes Glutamic Acid. Used in pumps such as Disetronic H-Tron, D-Tron and Minimed 500 series.

Lispro – Rapid Acting. Escherichia Coli.[85] B Chain alterations: 28 Proline becomes 28 lysine; 29 lysine becomes 29 Proline. Used in pumps such as Disetronic H-Tron, D-Tron and Minimed 500 series.

Regular – Zinc insulin crystal formation. It equilibrates from its normal hexamer (long-acting) form to monomer or dimeric form (short-acting) in order to pass through tissue.[78] Do not store in temperatures <2°C or >30°C. No direct sunlight.[AHFS, pg. 3253]

Neutral Protamine Hagedorn (AKA Isophane) or Protamine and regular insulin – biphasic absorption.

Isophane/NPH (Neutral Protamine Hagedorn - Each milliliter contains 100 units of insulin human & 0.35mg of protamine sulfate combined for crystal formation, 16mg of glycerin, 3.78mg of dibasic sodium phosphate, 1.6mg of metacresol, 0.65mg of phenol, zinc oxide content adjusted to provide 0.025mg zinc ion, and Water for Injection.[69]

Humalog U-100 contains insulin lispro 100 units, 16 mg glycerin, 1.88 mg dibasic sodium phosphate, 3.15 mg Metacresol, zinc oxide content adjusted to provide 0.0197 mg zinc ion, trace amounts of phenol, and Water for Injection. (Humalog 200 = lispro 200 units and Tromethamine.)[73]

Novolog: Each mL contains insulin aspart 100 units/mL, glycerin 16 mg/mL, phenol 1.50 mg/mL, metacresol 1.72 mg/mL, zinc 19.6 mcg/mL, disodium hydrogen phosphate dihydrate 1.25 mg/mL, sodium chloride 0.58 mg/mL and water for injection.[72]

Fiasp: Each mL contains 100 units of insulin aspart and the inactive ingredients: arginine (as L-arginine hydrochloride), USP (3.48 mg); disodium phosphate dihydrate, USP (0.53 mg); glycerol, USP (3.3 mg); metacresol, USP (1.72 mg); niacinamide, USP (20.8 mg); phenol, USP (1.50 mg); zinc (as zinc acetate), USP (19.6 mcg) and water for injection.[71]

Degludec – Ultra long-acting. S. Cerevisiae. B Chain alterations: 30 threonine is deleted; Addition f a glutamic acid side chain and a C16 fatty acid.[52]

Afrezza - Inhaled Insulin
Package Insert

Onset: 12 min. Peak: 35-55 min. Dur: 90min -4.5 hrs.
HbA_1C decrease 021%. FPG decrease – 25.
E. Coli recombinant insulin adsorbed onto carrier particles consisting of fumaryl diketopiperazine and polysorbate 80.
Albuterol will increase the AUC by 25% - monitor.
Sides: Acute bronchospasm, DKA, hypoglycemia, cough, throat pain, headache, diarrhea, productive cough, fatigue and nausea.
Due to the elevated risk of bronchospasm, prior to initiation a detailed medical history, physical exam and Forced Expiratory Volume (FEV1) must be performed to rule out asthma, COPD, infections or lung cancer.
DKA was three times higher with Afrezza than other insulin agents. Monitor blood and urine regularly.
This agent was not individually studied in renal or hepatic impairment.
Supplied as:
    4 units cartridge: 0.35mg insulin
    8 units cartridge: 0.7mg insulin
    12 units cartridge: 1 mg insulin

The package insert has a detailed conversion chart.

Anti-Hypoglycemic Agent/Glycogenolytic

Glucagon
AHFS 2016, Pgs.3296-3298

Available – only parenteral as stomach acids destroy glucagon as it does insulin. Available as the Glucagon Injection Kit for use in crash carts and from wholesalers. Patients should always carry immediate release sugar, like candy alongside this.
Given IM, IV or SQ.
Normal dose – 1mg. <=20Kg = 0.5mg. Also 20-30mcg/Kg
Once injected, may give another dose 15min later if still unresponsive. Then direct dextrose supplementation, especially in pediatrics, to restore hepatic glycogen supply and prevent secondary hypoglycemia.
Be aware of complications of cerebral hypoglycemia.
T1/2: 8-18 min IV. <45min IM. Peak: 30 min.
Dur: 60-90min.
Glucagon is a 29 amino acid. Histidine is the N-terminus and threonine is the C-terminus. It is prepared via recombinant DNA tech in E. Coli or S. Cerevisiae.

Mechanism of Action: Glucagon is a hormone synthesized and secreted by alpha-2 cells of the Islet of Langerhans and stimulates hepatic gluconeogenesis. Only effective if hepatic glycogen is available, so not effective in starvation states, adrenal insufficiency or chronic hypoglycemia where glycogen is depleted. Glucagon increases adenylate triphosphate to cyclic adenosine monophosphate in the liver, adipose and various other peripheral sites. cAMP then activates phosphorylase which then degrades glycogen to glucose.

Baroreceptor mechanisms secrete glucagon in response to low glucose concentrations or increased insulin levels to maintain homeostasis. The response depends upon the availability of glycogen and phosphorylases. Epinephrine administration will increase and attenuate the response due to vasoconstriction and sympathetic nervous system activation.

cAMP relaxes smooth muscle of the GI tract and reduces gastric and pancreatic secretions, and positive inotropic (force) and chronotropic (rate) activity of cardiac muscle. [Consider monitoring if antiarrhythmics, digoxin (positive inotrope/negative chronotrope) are used.] This in turn reduces blood pressure, plasma amine concentration, synthesis of protein and fat (glucose is preferred due to positive energy expenditure profile) and increases renal elimination of ionic molecules.[AHFS, pg.3297]

Sides: Rash, urticaria, hypotension and anaphylactic shock. Exogenous glucagon stimulates catecholamine release so blood pressure may increase.

Also used in Calcium channel blocker, beta blocker overdose at 50mcg/Kg over 1-2 min then 2-5mg/hr. Max 10mg in D5W.

Clinical Guidelines:
American diabetes Association
https://www.diabetes.org/diabetes

National Institute of Diabetes and Digestive and Kidney Diseases
https://www.niddk.nih.gov/health-information/diabetes

World Health Organization – Diabetes
https://www.who.int/news-room/fact-sheets/detail/diabetes

References:
1) Medscape. Accessed Nov. 7th, 2019. - https://reference.medscape.com/drug/onglyza-saxagliptin-999211#10
2) Bischoff, H. Bayer A.G. August 194 European Journal of Clinical Investigation. "Pharmacology of alpha-glucosidase Inhibition." Vol 24, Issue S3. https://doi.org/10.1111/j.1365-2362-1994.tb02249.x
3) Ramachandran, Anand "Pharmacology Recall." Lippincott, Williams and Wilkins. 2000.
4) Dipiro, et al. "Pharmacotherapy – A Pathophysiological Approach." 5th Edition. 2000. Pgs 1335-58.
5) Bedeker, Amrita. Advances in Applied Microbiology. 2010. Pgs.
6) Eberhard, Ritz. "Carbohydrate Metabolism in Kidney Disease." Nutritional Management of Renal Disease. 2013. https://www.researchgate.net/publication/281663801_Carbohydrate_Metabolism_in_Kidney_Disease_and_Kidney_Failure
7) Yvesheng, Dong, et al. "Intervention of Prediabetes by Flavanoids from Oroxylum Indicum." Bioactive Food as

Dietary Interventions for Diabetes. 2nd ed.
https://doi.org/10.1016/B978-0-12-813822-9.00036-9
8) AHFS Drug Information 2016. ASHP publishing. ISBN:978-1-58528-557-0. Pgs. 3188-3298. http://www.ahfsdruginformation.com
9) Drug Information Cards SFI Medical Publishing. 22nd Ed. 2006.
10) Glucosidases. Wikipedia. Accessed Nov. 4th, 2019. https://en.wikipedia.org/wiki.Glucosidases
11) Bansal V, Gassenhuber J, Phillips T, et al. Spectrum of mutations in monogenic diabetes genes identified from high-throughput DNA sequencing of 6888 individuals. *BMC Med*. 2017;15(1):213. Published 2017 Dec 6. doi:10.1186/s12916-017-0977-3
https://www.ncbi.nlm.nih.gov/pmc/articles/PMC5717832/
12) NIH - Monogenic Diabetes (Neonatal Diabetes Mellitus & MODY)
https://www.niddk.nih.gov/health-information/diabetes/overview/what-is-diabetes/monogenic-neonatal-mellitus-mody
13) NIH Website. Accessed Nov. 7th, 2019. *Type 1 Diabetes* https://ghr.nlm.nih.gov/condition/type-1-diabetes#genes
14) Montesanto A, Bonfigli AR, Crocco P, et al. Genes associated with Type 2 Diabetes and vascular complications. *Aging (Albany NY)*. 2018;10(2):178–196. http://doi.org/10.18632/aging.101375
15) AHFS Drug Information 2013. ASHP publishing. ISBN:978-1-58528-295-1. Pgs:3287-96 & 3190-3204. http://www.ahfsdruginformation.com
16) Briant L, Salehi A, Vergari E, Zhang Q, Rorsman P. Glucagon secretion from pancreatic α-cells [published correction appears in Ups J Med Sci. 2016 May;121(2):x]. *Ups J Med Sci*. 2016;121(2):113–119. http://doi.org/10.3109/03009734.2016.1156789
17) NIH website. Accessed Nov. 7th, 2019. *Dash diet* - https://www.nhlbi.nih.gov/health-topics/dash-eating-plan
18) US Department of Health and Human Services. National Institute of Diabetes and Digestive and Kidney Diseases. *Diabetes*. Accessed Nov. 4th, 2019.

https://www.niddk.nih.gov/health-information/kidney-disease/diabetes-insipidus
19) Cadel, S, Piesse, C, Pham, V, et al. Chapter 97 - Aminopeptidase B, *Handbook of Proteolytic Enzymes (3rd Ed.)* 2013:Pgs 473-479.https://doi.org/10.1016/B978-0-12-382219-2.00097-1.
20) Centers for Disease Control and Prevention. *Pregnancy*. Accessed Nov. 4th, 2019.
https://www.cdc.gov/pregnancy/diabetes-gestational.html
21) X. Li, Z.Q. Liu. "Pharmacogenetic Factors That Affect Drug Metabolism and Efficacy in Type 2 Diabetes Mellitus." *Drug Metabolism in Diseases*. Academic Press.2017, Pages 157-179 https://doi.org/10.1016/B978-0-12-802949-7.00007-9
22) Vella A. Mechanism of action of DPP-4 inhibitors--new insights. *J Clin Endocrinol Metab*. 2012;97(8):2626–2628. doi:10.1210/jc.2012-2396
https://www.ncbi.nlm.nih.gov/pmc/articles/PMC3410278/
23) Trapp S, Cork SC. PPG neurons of the lower brain stem and their role in brain GLP-1 receptor activation. *Am J Physiol Regul Integr Comp Physiol*. 2015;309(8):R795–R804.
doi:10.1152/ajpregu.00333.2015https://www.ncbi.nlm.nih.gov/pmc/articles/PMC4666945/
24) González-García I, Milbank E, Diéguez C, López M, Contreras C. Glucagon, GLP-1 and Thermogenesis. *Int J Mol Sci*. 2019;20(14):3445. Published 2019 Jul 13. doi:10.3390/ijms20143445
25) Lee, Young-Sun & Jun, Hee-Sook. (2016). Anti-Inflammatory Effects of GLP-1-Based Therapies beyond Glucose Control. *Mediators of Inflammation*. 2016. 1-11. 10.1155/2016/3094642.
https://www.researchgate.net/publication/299415845_Anti-Inflammatory_Effects_of_GLP-1-Based_Therapies_beyond_Glucose_Control
26) Tamez-Pérez HE, Quintanilla-Flores DL, Rodríguez-Gutiérrez R, González-González JG, Tamez-Peña AL. Steroid hyperglycemia: Prevalence, early detection and therapeutic recommendations: A narrative review. *World J*

Diabetes. 2015;6(8):1073–1081.
doi:10.4239/wjd.v6.i8.1073
https://www.ncbi.nlm.nih.gov/pmc/articles/PMC4515447/pdf/WJD-6-1073.pdf

27) Terrell, Jamie M. PharmD, and Jacobs, Tibbs F. PharmD, BCPS. Incretin Mimetics: Pros and Cons, and Emerging Agents in Diabetes Treatment. *American Journal of Managed Care.* 2013.
https://www.ajmc.com/journals/evidence-based-diabetes-management/2013/nov-dec-2013/incretin-mimetics-pros-and-cons-and-emerging-agents-in-diabetes-treatment?p=2

28) Seshadri, S, Rapaka, N, Prajapati, B, et al., 2019/06/19. Statins exacerbate glucose intolerance and hyperglycemia in a high sucrose fed rodent model. *Scientific Reports.* 2019;9(1) https://doi.org/10.1038/s41598-019-45369-8

29) Han KH. Functional Implications of HMG-CoA Reductase Inhibition on Glucose Metabolism. *Korean Circ J*. 2018;48(11):951–963.
https://doi.org/10.4070/kcj.2018.0307

30) Anderberg, R.H., Richard, J.E., et al. Glucagon-Like Peptide 1 and Its Analogs Act in the Dorsal Raphe and Modulate Central Serotonin to Reduce Appetite and Body Weight. *Diabetes* Apr 2017, 66 (4) 1062-1073;
https://doi.org/10.2337/db16-0755

31) Functional Anatomy of the Endocrine Pancreas http://www.vivo.colostate.edu/hbooks/pathphys/endocrine/pancreas/anatomy.html

32) Pacheco-López, Gustavo, Langhans, Wolfgang. *Handbook of Biologically Active Peptides* (2nd Ed). 2013, Pgs. 1111-7 https://doi.org/10.1016/B978-0-12-385095-9.00149-4

33) Liu, D., Jin, B., Chen, W. *et al.* Dipeptidyl peptidase 4 (DPP-4) inhibitors and cardiovascular outcomes in patients with type 2 diabetes mellitus (T2DM): a systematic review and meta-analysis. *BMC Pharmacol Toxicol* **20,** 15 (2019) doi:10.1186/s40360-019-0293-y
https://bmcpharmacoltoxicol.biomedcentral.com/articles/10.1186/s40360-019-0293-y

34) A Clinical Overview of DPP-4 Inhibitors for Type 2 Diabetes https://journalce.powerpak.com/ce/a-clinical-overview-of-dpp
35) *JAMA Dermatol.* 2018 Oct 1;154(10):1152-1158. doi: 10.1001/jamadermatol.2018.2352. https://www.ncbi.nlm.nih.gov/pubmed/30090931
36) Tomovic, K, Lazarevic, J, Kocic, G, Ilic, MD, Anderluh, M, Smelcerovic, A. Mechanisms and pathways of anti-inflammatory activity of DPP-4 inhibitors in cardiovascular and renal protection. *Med Res Rev.* 2019; 39: 404– 422. https://doi.org/10.1002/med.21513
37) Aldossari KK. Cardiovascular outcomes and safety with antidiabetic drugs. *Int J Health Sci (Qassim).* 2018;12(5):70–83.
38) Urakami T. New insights into the pharmacological treatment of pediatric patients with type 2 diabetes. *Clin Pediatr Endocrinol.* 2018;27(1):1–8. https://doi.org/10.1297/cpe.27.1
39) Faillie J, Yu OH, Yin H, Hillaire-Buys D, Barkun A, Azoulay L. Association of Bile Duct and Gallbladder Diseases With the Use of Incretin-Based Drugs in Patients With Type 2 Diabetes Mellitus. *JAMA Intern Med.* 2016;176(10):1474–1481. https://doi.org/10.1001/jamainternmed.2016.1531
40) Dina Halegoua-De Marzio, Victor J. Navarro, Hepatotoxicity of Cardiovascular and Antidiabetic Drugs. *Drug-Induced Liver Disease* (3rd Ed.) 2013:519-540. https://doi.org/10.1016/B978-0-12-387817-5.00029-7
41) Glimepiride. Medscape. Accessed Nov. 4th, 2019. https://reference.medscape.com/drug/amaryl-glimepiride-342707
42) Effects of glimepiride on HbA1c and body weight in Type 2 diabetes: results of a 1.5-year follow-up study. Weitgasser, Raimund et al. *Diabetes Research and Clinical Practice*, Volume 61, Issue 1, 13 - 19 DOI: 10.1016/S0168-8227(02)00254-1
43) Amaryl package insert. Accessed Nov. 8th, 2019. https://www.accessdata.fda.gov/drugsatfda_docs/label/2009/020496s021lbl.pdf

44) Micronized Glyburide package insert. Accessed Nov. 8th, 2019. https://www.accessdata.fda.gov/drugsatfda_docs/label/2011/020051s017lbl.pdf
45) Vicky Cheng and Sangeeta R. Kashyap, "Weight Considerations in Pharmacotherapy for Type 2 Diabetes," Journal of Obesity, vol. 2011, Article ID 984245, 9 pages, 2011. https://doi.org/10.1155/2011/984245.
46) Provilus, A., Abdallah, M., McFarlane, S. Weight gain associated with antidiabetic medications. *Therapy.* 8(2):113–120, MARCH 2011. DOI: 10.2217/thy.11.8
47) Pioglitazone package insert. Accessed Nov. 9th, 2019. https://www.fda.gov/drugs/postmarket-drug-safety-information-patients-and-providers/pioglitazone-marketed-actos-actoplus-met-duetact-and-oseni-information
48) Avandia package insert. Accessed Nov. 8th, 2019. https://www.fda.gov/media/75754/download
49) Pramlintide package insert. Accessed Nov 9th, 2019. https://www.azpicentral.com/symlin/symlin.pdf#page=1
50) Joanna McQueen, Pramlintide acetate, *American Journal of Health-System Pharmacy*, Volume 62, Issue 22, 15 November 2005, Pages 2363–2372, https://doi.org/10.2146/ajhp050341 https://academic.oup.com/ajhp/article-abstract/62/22/2363/5135438
51) https://www.accessdata.fda.gov/drugsatfda_docs/label/2011/021748s010lbl.pdf Package Insert Metformin. FDA website. Accessed Nov. 9th, 2019
52) Tresiba Package Insert. Accessed Nov. 9th, 2019. https://www.novo-pi.com/tresiba.pdf
53) Afrezza Package Insert. Accessed Nov. 9th, 2019. https://www.afrezza.com/pdf/Prescribing-Information-2019.pdf
54) Saxagliptin. Drugbank.ca website. Accessed Nov. 10th, 2019. https://www.drugbank.ca/drugs/DB06335
55) Alogliptin. Drugbank.ca website. Accessed Nov. 10th, 2019. https://www.drugbank.ca/drugs/DB06203

56) Jarvis, C.I., Cabrera, A., Charron, D. Alogliptin: A New Dipeptidyl Peptidase-4 Inhibitor for Type 2 Diabetes Mellitus. *Annals of Pharmacotherapy.* 2013.Vol.47; 11; 1532-9. https://doi.org/10.1177/1060028013504076
57) Thyroid Nodules. Cedars-Sinai.org website accessed Nov. 10th, 2019. https://www.cedars-sinai.org/health-library/diseases-and-conditions/t/thyroid-nodules.html
58) Linagliptin. Drugbank.ca. Accessed Nov. 10th, 2019. https://www.drugbank.ca/drugs/DB08882
59) Liraglutide. Drugbank.ca. Accessed Nov. 10th, 2019. https://www.drugbank.ca/drugs/DB06655
60) Exenatide. Drugbank.ca. Accessed Nov. 10th, 2019. https://www.drugbank.ca/drugs/DB01276
61) Ahmann AJ, Capehorn M, Charpentier G, et al. Efficacy and safety of once-weekly semaglutide versus exenatide ER in subjects with type 2 diabetes (SUSTAIN 3): a 56-week, open label, randomized clinical trial. Diabetes Care 2018;41:258–266. https://care.diabetesjournals.org/content/41/2/258.long
62) Semaglutide package insert. Accessed Nov. 10th, 2019. https://www.novo-pi.com/ozempic.pdf
63) Albiglutide package insert. Accessed Nov. 8th, 2019. https://www.gsksource.com/pharma/content/dam/GlaxoSmithKline/US/en/Prescribing_Information/Tanzeum/pdf/TANZEUM-PI-MG-IFU-COMBINED.PDF
64) Ertigliflozin. Medscape. Accessed Nov. 8th, 2019. https://reference.medscape.com/drug/steglatro-ertugliflozin-1000188
65) Ertigliflozin Package Insert. Accessed Nov. 10th, 2019. https://www.merck.com/product/usa/pi_circulars/s/steglatro/steglatro_pi.pdf
66) Dapagliflozin Package Insert. Accessed Nov. 9th, 2019. https://www.azpicentral.com/farxiga/farxiga.pdf#page=1
67) Ulrik Birk Lauridsen, Niels Juel Christensen, Jens LyngsøE, Effects of Nonselective and β-1-Selective Blockade on Glucose Metabolism and Hormone Responses during Insulin-Induced Hypoglycemia in Normal Man, *The Journal of Clinical Endocrinology &*

Metabolism, Volume 56, Issue 5, 1 May 1983, Pages 876–882, https://doi.org/10.1210/jcem-56-5-876
68) University of California at San Francisco. Diabetes Education Online. https://dtc.ucsf.edu/types-of-diabetes/type2/treatment-of-type-2-diabetes/medications-and-therapies/type-2-insulin-rx/calculating-insulin-dose/
69) Humulin N package insert. Lilly website. Accessed Nov. 10th, 2019. http://pi.lilly.com/us/HUMULIN-N-USPI.pdf
70) Humulin 70/30 package insert. Lilly website. Accessed Nov. 10th, 2019. http://uspl.lilly.com/humulin7030/humulin7030.html
71) Fiasp package insert. Accessed Nov. 10th, 2019. https://www.novo-pi.com/fiasp.pdf
72) Novolog package insert. Accessed Nov. 10th, 2019. https://www.novo-pi.com/novolog.pdf
73) Humalog package insert. Accessed Nov. 10th, 2019. https://pi.lilly.com/us/humalog-pen-pi.pdf
74) Woodward C, Pourmand A, Mazer-Amirshahi M. High dose insulin therapy, an evidence based approach to beta blocker/calcium channel blocker toxicity. *Daru*. 2014;22(1):36. Published 2014 Apr 8. https://doi.org/10.1186/2008-2231-22-36
75) Luther JM. Effects of aldosterone on insulin sensitivity and secretion. *Steroids*. 2014;91:54–60. https://doi.org/10.1016/j.steroids.2014.08.016
76) Mazaheri T, Sharifi F, Kamali K. Insulin resistance in hypothyroid patients under Levothyroxine therapy: a comparison between those with and without thyroid autoimmunity. *J Diabetes Metab Disord*. 2014;13(1):103. Published 2014 Oct 30. https://doi.org/10.1186/s40200-014-0103-4
77) Nakamura, K, Velho, G, Bouby, N (National Research Institute for Child Health and Development, Tokyo, Japan; Centre de Recherches des Cordeliers, Paris, France). Vasopressin and metabolic disorders: translation from experimental models to clinical use (Review Symposium). *J Intern Med* 2017; 282: 298–309. https://doi.org/10.1111/joim.12649

78) Melmed, S., Polonsky, K.S., Larsen, P.R., Kronenberg,H.M. *Williams Textbook of Endocrinology (13 Ed)*. Elsevier.2016, Pages 1451-1483 Author: Mark A. Atkinson. https://doi.org/10.1016/B978-0-323-29738-7.00032-0.
79) Standards of Medical Care in Diabetes—2019 Abridged for Primary Care Providers. American Diabetes Association. *Clinical Diabetes* Jan 2019, 37 (1) 11-34; https://doi.org/ 10.2337/cd18-0105
80) Emanuele, N.V., et al. Consequences of Alcohol Use in Diabetics. *Alcohol Health & Research World*. Vol. 22, No. 3, 1998. Pgs. 211-9. https://pubs.niaaa.nih.gov/publications/arh22-3/211.pdf
81) Sitagliptin package insert. Accessed Nov. 4th, 2019. https://www.merck.com/product/usa/pi_circulars/j/januvia/januvia_pi.pdf
82) Lixisenalide package insert. Accessed Nov. 13th, 2019. https://www.accessdata.fda.gov/drugsatfda_docs/label/2016/208471Orig1s000lbl.pdf
83) Dulaglutide package insert. Accessed Nov. 4th, 2019. https://www.accessdata.fda.gov/drugsatfda_docs/label/2017/125469s007s008lbl.pdf
84) Saccharomyces Cerevisiae. Kenyon University. Accessed Nov. 13th, 2019. https://microbewiki.kenyon.edu/index.php/Saccharomyces_cerevisiae
85) Escherichia coli. CDC website. Accessed Nov. 13th, 2019. https://www.cdc.gov/ecoli/index.html

www.ingramcontent.com/pod-product-compliance
Lightning Source LLC
Chambersburg PA
CBHW020620220526
45463CB00006B/2637